Super Sex at Sixty, Naturally!

Kenneth G Green

Contents

Important note:

Use the Glossary or a good dictionary for looking up the definitions of words you do not understand. Never go past any word you do not understand. The misunderstood word can cause confusion, boredom, and failure to learn and enjoy.

Super Sex at Sixty, Naturally!

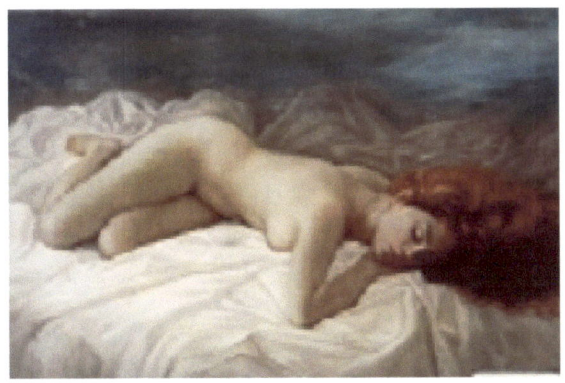

Age is not a barrier!

Some famous people are known for being sexy at sixty:

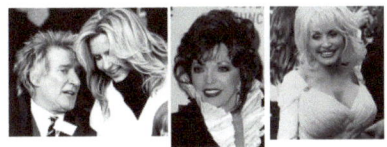

What is the key to Super Sex at Sixty? It begins with
Desire.

Part One:

Desire

Desire is everything to do with sex. Where there is no desire there is no sex. There are two kinds of desire; there is desire of the mind or spirit that some say is the only true reason for sex. But there is also physical desire, driven by hormones. Nature doesn't trust us to reproduce so most of the sexual machinery runs on automatic. Men have a constant urge for sex. They must always be ready to perform if the lady suddenly beckons. Women go through cycles though that make men redundant for half the month. This absence of desire in the female is matched by a frustrated desire in the male. No wonder that men have many wives in some cultures. However, by the age of sixty the problems of cycles and timing are a thing of the past. The couple gain a freedom to forget about reproduction and re-invent sex for pleasure. This treasure-trove of pleasure has one weak link: it depends on the body, which at sixty often shows signs of cracking under the strain. So our first project toward super sex at sixty is to re-create the body, naturally.

The Body

Sex at sixty can be better than sex at thirty. Firstly, at sixty there is no anxiety about falling pregnant. Secondly, there is more time because reaching orgasm is slower and so more satisfying. There is also less emphasis on orgasm as the only satisfaction of sex. At sixty, one has the time to experience more sensations than one did at thirty. One also has the time to look for new sensations and to learn new techniques that make the whole experience of sex a time of mutual enjoyment.

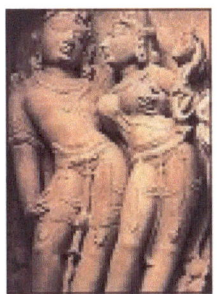

Why then does this ideal scenario not happen routinely to all sixty-year olds? The answer can be found in statistics of declining health that affects many over sixty: 60 percent of people aged 65 and over say they have a long-term condition, compared with 17 percent of those aged under 40. (Department of Health, Raising the profile of long term conditions care: A compendium of information, 2008) Without health there can be no enjoyment in sex. Health gives one important abilities; such as being able to move, think, communicate, and make energy. These abilities can be inherited but their presence in later life depends on what a person eats, and in particular, what a person has eaten for the previous forty years. How do we decide what is good food, or what food should be avoided, for a perfect sex experience?

Food and Sex

Simplified Science

Sex demands energy for success. Sex involves movement, sometimes more from one partner than the other and, as will be shown later, involving muscle action inside and around the vagina. We will look at foods that provide energy without creating unwanted fat.

What you eat can change your shape. Looking sexy is part of being sexy, and its easy to achieve, naturally.

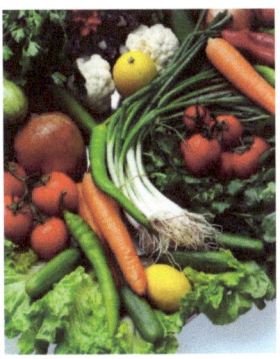

The correct diet will contain lots of salads with plenty of green leaves which contain natural chlorophyll, the plant substance that is a good source of magnesium. Lack of magnesium is the most common reason for lack of energy. Experiment with salads, there are lots of vegetable foods that can be eaten raw. Smoothies are a way to consume green leaves, simply add the leaves, for example, baby spinach to some fruit in a blender. You can also add wheatgrass powder or spirulina powder to increase the 'green' content. Spirulina also increases the pure protein content for repair of tissues and supply of amino acids for making hormones.

Energy

Energy is the end product of a sequence that converts food into a simple sugar called glucose. Grape sugar is glucose, and fruit sugar is fructose. These are very similar but not identical. Cane sugar (sucrose) is a compound of glucose and fructose. Your digestive system strives to convert all carbohydrate, starch, and compound sugars into simple glucose sugar. This is blood sugar. Glucose molecules contain carbon atoms held together by energy. The glucose is carried around the body in blood. Muscle cells which are energy hungry use enzymes to separate the carbon atoms and so release the energy. The enzymes will only work if there is magnesium in the blood. The whole sequence also needs vitamin B, and oxygen, which itself needs iron in the blood to attract it to a red blood cell. Who said chemistry was difficult?!

Plants are green because they contain chlorophyll and magnesium. Blood is red because it contains hemoglobin and iron and oxygen. Venous blood is blue because the oxygen in it is low, having been used up on its journey through muscle and organ cells.

Carbohydrates such as bread and potato are made from long chains of simple sugar (glucose) joined together. They can be a source of energy but carry the risk that they will create fat rather than energy. The fat leads to obesity as the body does its best to store the excess energy which it can't use. Here is some simple arithmetic: The average person can maintain a constant weight while consuming about 2,000 calories a day, but South Pole explorers pulling a sled can actually *lose* weight on 10,000 calories a day. It's a case of balancing the work output against the energy input. A high sugar and carbohydrate diet can easily add up to 3,000 calories per day. If your job or chores only need 2,000 calories a day then you will store the other 1,000 calories as fat. Remember that calories are just a measure of how much energy is stored in a food. When that energy is stored in the body it is called fat.

1lb (450 grams) of body fat is equivalent to about 3,000 calories. People who eat sugary or fatty snacks (think of a doughnut!) can easily consume an extra 500 calories a day. That could result in a new 1lb (450 grams) of body fat every week. You need energy for sex but not that sort of 'waist-full' energy. Remember, becoming obese may reduce your sex enjoyment and satisfaction.

Most people are sensitive to wheat, and do better without it. The same applies to dairy foods such as milk and cheese. There is a very large body of knowledge called 'nutrition' but it can be simplified for the majority of people by creating just two kinds of food: Those foods which should be eaten, and those which should be avoided. This basic plan will create the energy one needs for a satisfying sexual experience:

Eat as much green leaf and vegetable food as you like, but avoid potatoes. Eat cereal foods like oats, rice, quinoa, and millet, but avoid wheat flour in all its forms. Use 100 percent rye bread instead. Avoid sugar. Eat meat and chicken but remember that blood type A should avoid red meat, and blood type B should avoid chicken, soy, and rye. (Your blood creates anti-bodies, which can be harmful to your health, see the reference about blood types at the end.) Eat fish that has fins and bones: Avoid shark, whale, octopus and shellfish. Avoid dairy products from the cow. Use rice milk, or almond milk, or oat milk. Soy milk is not recommended because many people are sensitive to soy proteins. Rice milk comes in different flavours, and the Dream brand original organic is probably the best. Whatever your preference insist on organic.

Always have breakfast, such as oats, or millet, or quinoa, cooked as a porridge, or make a muesli from oats with fruit. Eggs and rye toast are good too! Having a hearty, but sugar-free, breakfast ensures that the blood sugar level stays in normal for most of the day.

A low blood sugar level is the most common cause of impulse nibbling on junk food snacks like chocolates or sticky buns, which then causes sudden peaks of high blood sugar. That in turn causes a release of insulin which turns the sugar to fat if it is not immediately required for energy. Caffeine from coffee or cola has the same effect, so avoid it.

Diabetes is simple and everyone should understand it. There are two basic kinds of Diabetes: Diabetes Type 1 begins when one can no longer make insulin. This results in blood sugar levels being too high and not being able to make energy from the sugar. Diabetes Type 2 is caused by insulin resistance where body tissues fail to respond appropriately to insulin. Again, the blood sugar level is raised. This condition is often associated with obesity, and lack of energy. The third condition is not diabetes but related: If one has the ability to continually make insulin despite having too much sugar in the diet, the insulin triggers fat cells to make more fat. That is how some people can be obese but not diabetic.

Diabetic blood glucose tests have been shown to return to normal levels in as little as 30 days through strict diet control. The secret is to rebuild the quality of the blood through the diet. This means increasing the amount and variety of salads every day, and totally eliminating sugar and other refined foods. The B vitamins and the minerals may need supplementing as well as obtaining a regular dose of natural sunlight. Lack of Vitamin D has been shown to be associated with raised blood sugar levels.

Lack of Vitamin D is also to blame for strokes, those damaging moments when a part the brain is starved of oxygen. It is often caused by a bleeding in the brain, but can also be caused by a clot that blocks a blood vessel. Scientists at the University of Alabama discovered that lack of sunlight is positively associated with stroke: the more sunlight the fewer strokes. The scientists also commented on the poor wisdom of avoiding all sunlight. In other words, get a natural tan to avoid premature death, or disability, from a stroke!

What can one add to a diet to improve the food value and create more energy? Is it really necessary to supplement good food with vitamin tablets?

Supplements

Vitamins. Minerals. Oils.

Energy, health, and super-sex can be achieved naturally by food designed for health. Sometimes though the food available does not contain enough minerals or vitamins and needs supplementing. People have different body structures, and different levels of metabolism, so need different quantities of nutrients. Even racing horses get supplements to make them better racers.

The most common supplement taken is probably vitamin C. This is useful for protecting the heart as much as protecting oneself from infection. In days gone by sailors often suffered from a disease called scurvy. It is caused by a deficiency of vitamin C and its symptoms include anaemia and rough skin. Skin contains a network of connective tissue called collagen; lack of vitamin C allows collagen to break down and body tissues to lose strength and elasticity. Blood vessels also contain collagen so begin to disintegrate if vitamin C is missing. Dr. Matthias Rath a former director of Cardiovascular Research at the Linus Pauling Institute in Palo Alto, California, discovered a direct link between lack of vitamin C and cardio-vascular heart disease. He observed that dogs don't naturally suffer heart attacks, because dogs make their own vitamin C. The sailors who had scurvy usually died of internal bleeding. Limes cured that, but so would lots of other fresh fruit and vegetables. Vitamin C is so important to health that it is worth the effort to take a daily supplement of at least 500mg of Vitamin C. Lack of vitamin C can cause tiredness and no enthusiasm for sex!

The next most supplemented vitamins are the B complex group. Vitamin B1 is needed for energy, B3 for hormones, and B6 for moods. Not forgetting B12 for iron absorption (which leads back to energy), and B5 for nerve-to-muscle communication and fat metabolism in the production of energy. The body needs just a few milligrams of vitamin B daily but suffers badly if the B vitamins are lacking. Many mental symptoms are associated with vitamin B deficiency. Often the cause of the B deficiency is simply a lack of the essential minerals needed to activate the B vitamins. Iron, zinc, copper, magnesium, manganese, and sulphur are all needed at some point in the chemistry of the body.

High blood sugar is sometimes caused by lack of chromium which is needed to activate insulin (one of the hormones). Chromium was identified as the active ingredient in GTF, the 'glucose tolerance factor', in 1959. Low levels of GTF lead to mood swings, lack of sex drive, and tiredness. Insulin, like thyroxin, is a controlling hormone of our metabolism; it not only controls blood sugar levels and many other aspects of carbohydrate breakdown and storage, but also directs much of the metabolism involving fat, protein and energy.

Because insulin requires chromium in order to function properly, this trace element has significant biological effects in the body. Chromium deficiency may contribute to some of the manifestations of obesity, diabetes, abnormal blood fats, high blood pressure and coronary artery disease. Too much fat in the blood combined with high blood pressure and a weak heart is a recipe for trouble. In other words, all the reasons for a failed sex life! To prevent chromium deficiency eat some of the following foods everyday:

Some food sources of chromium:
Brewers Yeast, Mushrooms, Beef, Organ Meats, Broccoli, Parsnips, Lamb Chops, Grape juice, Potatoes, Garlic, Basil, Orange juice, Turkey breast, Whole Spelt or Rye Bread, Apple, Banana, Blueberries, Strawberries, Green beans, Eggs, Molasses.

Vitamin C and vitamin B3 (niacin) will increase absorption of chromium which is stored in the liver, spleen, soft tissue, and bone. Diets high in simple sugars can increase chromium excretion in the urine. Or, in basic terms, sugar causes a loss of chromium in the urine. Infection, acute exercise, pregnancy and lactation, as well as stress increase chromium losses and can lead to deficiency, especially if chromium intakes are already low.

The function of sex depends on two things: Energy and hormones.

There are four key nutrients which are needed in the production of these hormones: Zinc, vitamin B3, magnesium, and vitamin B6. Of course there should also be protein which is easily supplied from beans, nuts, eggs, fish, fowl, and meat. Also fats which will come from the same foods. The carbon atoms that are found in sugars are also found in fats and oils. Hard fats have longer chains of carbon atoms, and liquid oils have shorter carbon chains. Olive oil is one of the best sources of dietary fat and is of course a component of the healthy Mediterranean diet. Sunshine is not a vitamin but we can't live without it. Sunshine on the skin converts pre-vitamin D (a cholesterol molecule) to vitamin D (a hormone and vitamin).

Some vitamin supplements function better in their active form. These are able to perform as co-factors for the enzymes that need them. See the glossary for extra definitions of these words.

Hormones

What are hormones, and how do they impact on sex?

Hormones are substances produced in one part of the body that then travel directly via the blood to affect another part of the body. Some hormones also behave as neuro-transmitters, meaning that the hormone travels directly along nerve pathways to cause an effect, usually in the brain. The pineal gland in the brain produces the substance called dopamine, which as a hormone affects sexual moods, and as a neuro-transmitter affects the control of movement through muscles. If your dopamine was lacking you would probably not be interested in sex, nor would you be able to perform the act of intercourse.

Some of the hormones are called steroid hormones. These are a group which include testosterone and estrogen, as well as progesterone cortisol and vitamin D. These hormones are all made from cholesterol, which shows that not everything about cholesterol is bad! The conversion process requires the active form of vitamin B3, (called NADPH). Without this molecule the body has difficulty converting cholesterol into the hormones. The second step for these hormones involves the mineral zinc. Lack of zinc is frequently seen as stretch marks on the skin, usually around the waist, buttocks, upper arms, and breasts, or as white spots on the finger nails. Zinc is found in protein foods, like meat, fish, and chicken. It is also found to a lesser degree in plant proteins like nuts and beans.

Oxytocin is a brain chemical (neuro-transmitter) known for its role as a pregnancy hormone, promoting contractions and aiding breastfeeding. But that is not the whole picture: During the male orgasm, the production of oxytocin helps produce contractions of the prostrate and seminal glands. During the female orgasm the immediate effect of oxytocin are uterine contractions that transport the sperm to the ova. Oxytocin is also related to the bonding that occurs between couples having sex. Stimulating the nipple, and its areola, will produce oxytocin hence couples touching and sucking each others nipples during foreplay and intercourse will create a sensation of bonding and lead to greater satisfaction from sex. From a nutrition viewpoint the action of oxytocin requires the minerals magnesium and manganese. Magnesium is particularly found in green leafy foods and nuts and seeds. Manganese is found in mustard greens, kale, chard, raspberries, pineapple, strawberries, romaine lettuce, collard greens, spinach, garlic, summer squash, grapes, turnip greens, eggplant, brown rice, blackstrap molasses, maple syrup, cloves, cinnamon, thyme, black pepper, and turmeric.

Thyroid hormone (thyroxin), to be produced in the body, needs iodine. Sources of iodine include: Asparagus, Dulse, Garlic, Kelp, Lima beans, Mushrooms, Seafood, Sea salt and Fortified Salt, Seaweed, Sesame seeds, Soybeans, Spinach, Summer squash, Swiss chard, and Turnip greens. Iodine can also be taken as a liquid tincture of iodine. The dose depends on the degree of iodine deficiency, and must be calculated by the therapist. The best way to get iodine is to ensure that the soil contains iodine before planting vegetables. Fertilising soil with seaweed is a simple solution.

Why is thyroxin so important? Because it provides the rate at which things happen in the body. Thyroxin controls metabolism, and that controls how fast you can make and use energy. No thyroxin means no sex. Symptoms of under-active thyroid commonly include: tiredness, weight gain, constipation, aches, feeling cold, dry skin, lifeless hair, fluid retention, mental slowing, and depression. Other symptoms include: hoarseness of voice, loss of sex drive, carpal tunnel syndrome (pains and numbness in the hand), and memory loss. Does that sound like an ideal sexual partner? Could there be a simple solution? Some say that the answer lies in raw vegan foods.

Raw Food for Sex?

In the beginning sex and eating were both simple; we eat natural food to stay alive, and had sex on impulse. But then we humans began tampering with food. First we began cooking our food, then we refined it, for example, making white sugar and white bread. In both actions the food lost quality, and we lost vitality, energy, and sex enjoyment. Nature intended us to get all the vitamins and minerals from our food, which is unfortunately not possible anymore - unless you happen to be a health-nut and eat everything raw and organic. Maybe the 'Raw Fooders' are not so nutty after all! Perhaps that is the way we should all go – eat raw and organic. Only if that is not possible should you then take supplements. If your sex enjoyment is important to you look up the story of the Hippocrates Institute which is in Florida, USA. This is a clinic that uses only organic raw food for clients and cures any 'un-wellness' that comes their way, including loss of sex function. This raw vegan organic approach is a unique way to supply the missing vitamins and minerals, and avoids the three common culprits: bread, dairy, and meat. In fact the 'Raw Fooders' avoid anything from an animal. Only babies are allowed milk, and then only from a human breast. The rest of the diet is vegan. If it solves your sex problems why argue with it?

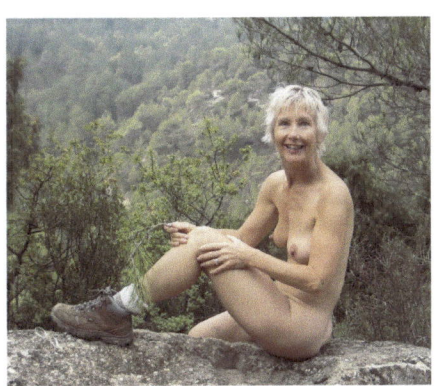

One aspect of natural living is sunlight. We make vitamin D from sunlight in our skin then convert it into a powerful hormone in the liver and the kidneys. We call the hormone form, vitamin D3, so as to distinguish it from the pre-hormone form in the skin. Vitamin D3 controls the movement of calcium and the creation and maintenance of bone. (Eggs have thin egg-shells when the hen lacks Vitamin D3 or sunshine.) Vitamin D3 also controls the action of many genes that are responsible for health and the prevention of cancer and diabetes. There is so much research in progress on vitamin D3 that scientists meet every four years in a different country to share information just on vitamin D3. No part of the body can function properly with this vitamin-hormone yet we seem to actively do things that reduce our chances of making the vitamin D3 naturally. For instance we avoid going outdoors into the sunlight in case we get sunburn, or worse still, skin cancer. For this reason we cover ourselves in sunblock crème, or wear clothes to hide the skin. Yet research suggests that vitamin D3 actually protects against cancer. Mothers who are deficient in vitamin D3 will give birth to babies who are also deficient as will be the mother's breast milk thereby depriving the baby of a vital nutrient. The result can be rickets, a bone disease of calcium deficiency, or brain inflammation, or autism.

The Medical University of Graz in Austria, published a study showing that testosterone levels are directly associated with vitamin D levels and that testosterone levels vary with the seasons, in concert with vitamin D levels. Symptoms of low testosterone levels in women include: Loss of sexual desire; tiredness and fatigue; mood changes; sleep disturbances; and reduced motivation. One can conclude that for a healthy satisfying sex life, one needs vitamin D3.

Sunlight is the natural source of vitamin D3 but it depends on what time of the year, what time of the day, and where on the planet one is sunbathing! To make it easy for people to know how strong the sunlight is in any particular place, the weather experts always add a line to weather forecasts showing what the expected sun-strength will be. This is called the Ultra-Violet Index, or UV Index. In Florida, USA, this reaches a maximum of 14, while in Britain it reaches a maximum of 7. Suntanning begins at UV index 3 or 4, which is about average for Britain. As a rule of thumb, if one's shadow is longer than one's height then there will not be enough intensity in the sunlight to make vitamin D. The best time to make vitamin D is of course in summer between 10 am and 2 pm which is also the best time to get sunburn so common sense is needed. If one starts tanning at the beginning of summer the skin adjusts to the gradually increasing amount of UV light. The wrong way is to jet off to a hot country and start suddenly exposing oneself to hours of blazing hot sunshine. Treat a hot country as you would a sun tanning bed; just a few minutes each day gradually increasing the length of exposure. In direct sunshine one needs to turn pink to reach safe maximum light absorption for making vitamin D. Cover up before you turn red! Doing this every day leads to a safe tan and better long term protection against sunburn.

Vitamin A protects the skin against sun damage, but it also reduces the benefits of vitamin D3. For anyone not accustomed to the sun I would suggest taking a daily dose of vitamin A until the skin is fully tanned then stop the vitamin A supplement. Normal healthy food contains pro-vitamin A substances (like beta-carotene) that the liver converts into vitamin A. These are found in the dark green, orange, and red vegetables and fruits. Vitamin D plays a part in brain chemistry and has been studied in relation to depression. Vitamin D appears to protect against depression, and since sexual enjoyment is not possible when you are depressed, it makes sense to supplement with Vitamin D3, or get more exposure to sunshine!

Supplements can be important for those people who are unable to efficiently convert their vitamins into the active forms as required to make hormones. Hormones, moods, and mind are closely related, so this is a good point to think about the functioning of the mind: What is the connection between mind and sexual satisfaction?

Part Two

Mind and Memory
The Creation of Sex

What is the mind? Where is the mind?

Wanting sex or not wanting sex are both thoughts. Thoughts originate in the mind, so we had better find out more about the mind. The mind is not to be confused with the Being or the Soul or the Spirit. You have a mind but you are a Being. Despite beliefs to the contrary, the fact is that after death you simply stay on earth and start again with a new body. Your Beingness is uninterrupted, or in other words, you really are immortal. As a Being you think, which leads to a decision, which one could imagine as a future action of some sort. For example, you think about sex and therefore decide to have intercourse or coitus as the medical fraternity like to call it. It is going to happen in the near or far future, but your thinking has set the wheels of action in motion. The problem arises if you forget that you made a decision or that you wanted something in the future. Sometimes we even have negative thoughts which work their way into a decision, such as, 'I am going to be late for work'. That might have been valid on one day, about twenty years ago, but is not valid nor desirable today or tomorrow or any other day in the future. Simply recalling (remembering) that decision will give one the opportunity to keep or remove that thought. In other words one can choose what to think and what to be effect of. You don't have to have sex tonight just because you thought it was a good idea two weeks ago. One doesn't have to always fail at sex just because one had a bad experience forty years ago. If you listen to people you will notice how negative their speech can be: 'I can never start a conversation', 'I am always tripping up', 'I never find the bargains'. 'I always say the wrong thing'. These individuals give themselves a controlling command. They create their own discomfort!

The mind, on the other hand, has a different function and structure. The mind is closely connected with the body in the sense that hormones and nutrition and injury can alter the relationship between Being and Mind. The Being may wish to be well and happy, but an injury containing pain and unconsciousness may alter the mind so that the Being is unhappy and sick. This is the basis of psycho-somatic illness. (Psyche: spirit, Soma: body). The mind is a link between the Being and the body. Problems with sex? Look for pictures in the mind that contain sex and pain. During an injury the mind can record perceptions such as sound, sight, and touch. The mind will remember the time of day, temperature, motion, sounds of voices, and sensations of pain. The mind stores these in the subconscious so that they can be used again sometime in the future. The reason is: Survival. You know that getting injured and especially getting injured and unconscious is potentially a non survival situation. These days we have emergency medical teams that can bring one back from the dead with electric shocks to the heart, transfusions, and a surgeon's steady hand. But it wasn't always like that. Our genes and our mental architecture are anchored in the past, in a way that is more suited to an animal than an intelligent Being. The events of a life threatening event may re-occur, in which case your mind would rather not be there. This is why the mind records and remembers everything about such an event so as to recognise it again in the future. If you fell off a horse and were rendered unconscious your mind would rather you stayed away from horses in the future. Subsequently, being near horses may bring on a dislike for horses, or if that didn't work, you would get pains where you had them as a result of falling off a horse. Your mind calculates that pain will achieve the goal of keeping you safe by being unable to ride horses!

Not all the mind behaves in this fashion, but that small bit that clings to our animal genes from the past can cause havoc in someone's life. Because babies in the womb are easily injured by accidents that mother has, there are plenty of opportunities for unpleasant memories to be laid in even before baby is born. Birth itself is a moment of unconsciousness for the baby accompanied by a good dose of pain. If mother vocalises her discomfort with plenty of shrieking and cursing then that soundtrack is included in the baby's memory. All that is associated with the vagina. Later it is possible to restimulate that memory and have that Being experience discomfort and dislike. It is a perfect combination for ruining sex. Because language is a modern device, compared to our prehistoric origin, mental memories can be completely confused by words. For example, a paramedic arrived on the scene of a minor accident where the injured person was in a dazed state. The paramedic shouted 'don't move!' just in case there were any broken bones. However, the effect on this patient was to create a time-warp where the person stayed in that moment of time for a number of years. The mind was obeying a command not to move. The mind isn't always logical or rational!

So, the first rule of being able to enjoy sex is to understand your mind and how it functions. The second rule is to understand the link between what you eat and what happens in your mind. The brain is fed directly from your blood. Food is digested in the stomach and small intestine from where it travels to the liver. The liver performs a hundred actions on the food going through it, including activating vitamins, storing sugar for future energy, and making cholesterol. The liver makes and uses enzymes. In particular the wonderful enzyme called 'CP450' that removes toxins from your blood, both from the outside world and the interior world of your metabolism. Drugs, medical and recreational, and alcohol are specially targeted by CP450! Some people have irrational reasons for eating junk food or not eating at all (anorexia). They become victims of their brain chemistry because the brain can't think if it can't make energy. Moods can alter if brain chemicals such as serotonin or dopamine, are in short supply. Depression may result, and consequently no desire for sex, or no enjoyment from sex. Sugar is a factor in the mind too: Glucose is the main fuel in the brain but if the blood glucose level is too high the pancreas will secrete extra insulin into the blood to remove the excess sugar from the blood. Sometimes this glucose-insulin response is too active and the blood sugar level is brought down too far. The result is a malfunctioning brain with symptoms of mood swings, migraines, tiredness, sugar craving, and irrational behaviour. A nutritionally dysfunctional brain loses all interest in sex. Also remember 'Cooper's Droop' – the loss of male erection through consuming too much alcohol. Could medication have a similarly adverse effect on sex?

Medication

Serotonin-enhancing anti-depressants (SSRIs), have been reported to blunt the emotions, including the elation of romance, and suppress obsessive thinking, a critical component of romance. These antidepressants also inhibit orgasm, clitoral stimulation, penile erection, and deposit of seminal fluid (ejaculation). Seminal fluid contains dopamine and norepinephrine, oxytocin and vasopressin, testosterone and estrogen. (See the glossary for definitions of these words) Without an orgasm, men lose the ability to send courtship signals. Too much serotonin can dampen sexual desire and excitement. (From a study published in 2002, by anthropologist Helen Fisher PhD of Rutgers University.)

Dopamine and Oxytocin (see the glossary) also play an integral role in sex. Daily bonding behaviours can make your partner look better and better—at least to you. This is why daily affection, with less orgasm can strengthen your bond with your mate. Ordinary intercourse, with its emphasis on sexual satiation, causes separation and estrangement between partners and chaos in society. In some alternative cultures it is believed that making love without conventional orgasm, results in improved health, greater harmony between partners, increased moral strength, and even a decrease in cravings and impulsive behaviour. Scientists think that this kind of lovemaking balances our neurochemistry, keeping us off the extremes of intense attraction (leading to sexual overdose and boredom) followed by aversion or separating behaviour. It also strengthens emotional bonds between partners, because an exchange of 'giving care and attention behaviour' is a subconscious signal to our brains to bond emotionally.

Certain surgeries and many medications, such as blood pressure medications, antihistamines, antidepressants and acid-blocking drugs, can affect sexual function.

It is important not to suppress the brain chemistry of sex by taking drugs for another condition seemingly unrelated.

Antidepressants are the medicines most frequently implicated in causing sexual dysfunction but there are at least twenty different categories of medicine that adversely affect sexual function. Always look for the cause of your health problem. If arthritis prevents enjoyment of sex, then taking drugs for arthritis may worsen the sex problem. Find relief for the arthritis through correct diet and nutritional supplements, and your sexual satisfaction will also improve. Its not 'all in the mind', but chemicals created by the body, and chemical drugs, do affect the mind which in turn affects your sexual satisfaction. The key may be as simple as understanding the problem.

Understanding

Now that you have a picture of how the mind works its time to go back to the real you, the Being that animates the body and owns the mind.

You have a huge range of 'Beingness' starting with emotion. Your emotional possibilities cover all the scale from joyfully happy down to apathy and death. In between you will find boredom, conservatism, antagonism, anger, fear, pain, and grief. Between these there are even finer levels. Each emotion is accompanied by physical characteristics as well as chemical characteristics. Emotions are part of a scale of Affinity, which is the degree of liking someone or something, or the willingness to share space with someone or something. Sex requires you to share a space with someone, and to like that person. Of course there can be forced sex but that would be quite low on the emotional scale. Rather, we are interested in a relationship of two people who want, and enjoy, each other's company. The higher up the scale each person is the more enjoyment there will be from sex. For sex to be perfect the chemistry of the sexual organs needs to be perfect too. Being angry turns on the flow of adrenalin which stops the secretion of lubricant mucus. If one is chronically angry sex will dry up. Fear has a similar effect. Being chronically anxious is not helpful! You want to be happy and cheerful, or at worst, mildly interested, anything lower down the scale gets in the way of fully enjoyable sex. At the bottom of the scale is sadism, pain, and punishment, a sickness of the mind reflected into the body.

You and your sexual partner have to agree on what you are about to do. How does one come to an agreement about something as important as sex? Through communication! Talk to each other, say what you like and don't like. It might be that you have hidden memories in your subconscious mind that are influencing your attitude toward sex, but if you don't discuss this how will your partner ever know? The combination of communication, agreement, and affinity create an understanding. Lacking one of these is likely to lead to a misunderstanding, and – no sex!

Communication is more than just talking to somebody. It is looking at someone and being there for them to see that you are talking to them. It is having an intention of passing an idea from you to them, and for the other person to actually hear what you said. Always get a response to your communication, otherwise how do you know that the other person heard you? Did they actually get the message? If you asked your loved one whether he or she would like some nooky and you got a negative answer, you might feel rejected. But your loved one may have not heard or understood the word you used. What if they thought you had said 'new key', and in fact had wondered what you were on about but thought it best not to say so? That would be a simple misunderstanding with sad consequences, all because you failed to make sure that they had heard you!

Part Three

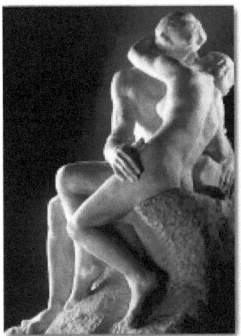

Techniques

This is where most people start. What position shall we use? Boredom creeps in to routine habits, and enjoyment diminishes.

But that could be the result of not 'creating' during lovemaking. Orgasm is a goal, but not the only goal. Pleasure is a bigger goal.

The Karma Sutra from India did much to show the inhibited English that there was much pleasure to be had through variation of position during sexual intercourse.

There are numerous other books similar to the Karma Sutra which demonstrate different positions to use during sex and foreplay, but we are looking for something more satisfying than simply a new position.

That font of pleasure is found in the G-Spot (The Gräfenberg Spot). This is often described as a sensitive spot inside the vagina behind the pubic bone. The G-Spot is part of the clitoris, which will be described further on. By inserting a finger (well lubricated with KY Jelly or similar) into the vagina this spot can be stimulated to give pleasure, both as a sensation of touch, and as a powerful orgasm inducer.

There is also another way, and that is to use the G-Spot to train the pelvic floor muscles to contract against the G-Spot. This can be used for self-stimulation, or during intercourse to squeeze against the erect penis inside the vagina. Both parties get intense pleasure from this action.

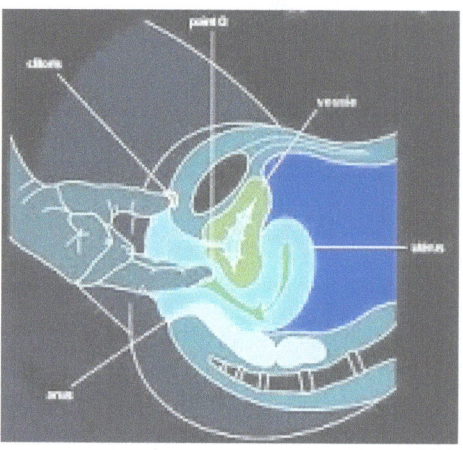

The first step is to find the G-Spot, then gently rub one or two fingers in a 'come hither' fashion in the vagina against the anterior wall which separates the vagina from the bladder. The keyword is *gently!* The next step is for the pelvic muscles to press against the rubbing finger. This takes some practice but is well worth the time invested. Eventually it is possible to squeeze at will with or without the finger there. When starting on this exercise it is necessary for a partner to do the G-Spot stroking while the lady learns what to do to make the muscle contract in the right place. As soon as the fingers feel a squeeze one acknowledges this in order to create a feedback loop. This way the one doing the squeezing learns and re-enforces the pelvic muscle action. The stimulating fingers will actually ache and feel bruised after about five to ten minutes of doing the exercise correctly, but its all in a good cause!

With more positive feedback like this a woman can soon learn to control both the perineal muscle which runs from side to side, and the pubo-coccygeus muscle which runs from front to back. Dr Kegel (see below) described the pubo-coccygeus as 'the most versatile muscle in the entire human body'. The pelvic floor is made in two halves, with a divider midway between the anus and the vaginal entrance.

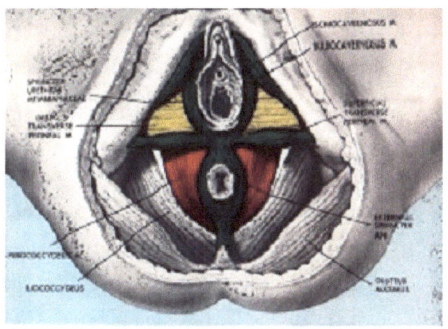

The PC muscle, (pubococcygeus) muscle, is actually a sling of muscles that support the pelvic floor and surround the internal genitalia. These muscles are involved in

urination (when you stop yourself from peeing in mid-stream, you're using your PC muscles). The PC muscles are also involved in orgasm, and many women find that doing regular exercises to strengthen the pelvic muscles changes the way their sexual response feels. Exercises that strengthen the PC muscles are usually referred to as Kegel exercises (Arnold H. Kegel, M.D., F.A.C.S. Assistant Professor of Gynaecology University of Southern California School of Medicine 1948).

It is possible to tone the PC muscle without knowing anything about the G-spot. Remember that Kegel started his famous pelvic floor exercises in 1948 but the G-spot was only observed in 1952.

An important physical characteristic of the vagina is that the PC muscle surrounds the opening of the vagina and covers the pelvic floor. This muscle may be lacking in firmness in some women. Like any other muscle, the PC muscle needs exercise to keep it in its best condition. A series of exercises were developed by Dr. Kegel for women with the common problem of urinary incontinence. These women would expel urine when they sneezed or coughed and these exercises were designed to tighten the PC muscle, and help them retain the urine. Many gynaecologists recommend these exercises routinely to women after childbirth in order to develop vaginal and rectal muscle support. Women who conscientiously carry out these exercises find they develop better control of their bowels and bladder. In addition to this they may also discover that the vagina, through these exercises, regains its former tightness for satisfying intercourse.

A welcome side effect was noted in that some of the women who followed Dr. Kegel's advice reported that after about six weeks of practicing the exercises they experienced increased pleasure during sexual intercourse. and better sensitivity in the vaginal area. In addition, strengthening the PC muscle helps reduce spontaneous urination with orgasm.

This exercise tightens the vagina over time so that there is more contact with the penis during intercourse. Like any other muscle in the body the pubic muscles must be regularly used to maintain the tone. In the beginning the pubic exercises should be practised daily to achieve condition, then maintained at least once or twice a week. Because it is such pleasure most couples have no problem finding the time to enjoy the 'vaginal-gym' workout!

A more indirect approach is to massage the female genitalia every morning on waking. Women love to be touched from head to toe and specially while they are still wrapped in the warm embrace of a duvet. On waking gently massage the face by slowly rubbing little circles on the cheeks, around the eyes, ears, nose, and mouth. These areas are rich in acupuncture points for vital systems in the body, including the hormonal systems. Gradually work down towards the neck, shoulders, and breasts, always been gentle. Remember that this is a sexual arousal massage, not a Swedish remedial massage! When you reach the pubic area rub the vulva between finger and thumb, slowly, being careful not to pinch the delicate tissues. Let a finger slip into the edge of the vagina so that you can rub the vagina and vulva together. At the lower end of the vagina are the Bartholin's glands, that when stimulated will arouse the whole clitoris and the vagina. Near the upper end of the vagina are the Skene's glands which connect the G-Spot to the urethra (the urinary outlet). It is thought by some that Skene's gland causes the female ejaculation. While massaging the vulva and these glands you may feel moisture start to flow. Let your fingers move to the clitoris and with a feather light touch rub across the shaft until it is firm and erect within its sheath and hood. Now is the time to enjoy intercourse.

Central to this exercise and satisfying sex, is the clitoris. Most of the vagina and vulva are part of the clitoris. The external female genitalia is known as the 'Vulva', while the internal female genitalia is known as the 'Vagina'. In the next chapter we'll look at the clitoris in a bit more detail.

Anatomy

The Clitoris

This female organ is mostly hidden behind muscle at the front of the female pelvis. The word clitoris comes from Greek meaning 'little hill'. The visible part of the clitoris is only one tenth of the whole organ. The vaginal wall is, in fact, a part of the clitoris. During stimulation the entire clitoris swells up with blood much like the penis does. The clitoris undergoes an erection too and the tip of the clitoris, called the glans, may become visible beyond the hood that normally covers it. Sometimes the visible clitoris is large enough to take on the appearance of a small penis.

The aroused clitoris takes on a different shape due to engorgement with blood. During sexual arousal, the intricate chambers of these tissues fill with blood which is then trapped by valves, and the entire clitoris enlarges and changes dramatically. The glans and shaft become erect and maintain their positions until resolution. Underneath, the muscles are taut and contract in response to sexual stimulation.

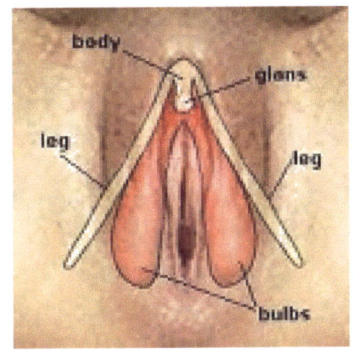

After arousal, when the orgasm has subsided, the clitoris returns to its resting state.

Where libido is low or absent, a gentle touch and movement across the clitoris will arouse it and set in motion a chain of other arousal actions leading to pleasurable sensation. Because one doesn't feel 'in the mood' doesn't mean that one can't get in the mood for sex. A woman may think that she is not interested, until she is touched in the right way. Sometimes this may just be a kiss on the neck, or a warm hand on a breast. Othertimes it might be a gentle finger on the clitoris that triggers the sexual response.

A study conducted by sociologists Cameron and Fleming in the USA asked a representative sampling of Americans of both sexes—ranging in age from 18 to 55—to rank in order 22 pleasurable activities on a five-point scale. In the 40 to 55 age group, sex drops far down the scale. Males listed it behind family, in joint second place with nature, but females in this group listed sex 15th, behind mundane activities such as sleeping, attending church, watching TV, and housework.

Could this mean that a middle-aged American housewife would rather clean house than have sex?

One possible explanation is simply that women do not enjoy sex, and that the older they get the less satisfaction they get from sex. By the time a woman gets to be sixty she might be turned off sex completely. There are many possible reasons for this, and it may account for many divorces too, but one explanation is that circumcised men are causing pain in the vagina by over-thrusting. Because the foreskin has more nerve endings it allows the penis to develop the orgasm with shorter strokes. It also prevents dryness in the vagina. A circumcised man has to learn to feel the subtle sensations around the top of the penis beneath the glans, and the ring of tissue that used to attach the foreskin to the shaft of the penis just below the head. The man's movements must be gentle and rhythmical without withdrawing the penis (that allows air into the vagina and has a drying effect). Circumcised men should not be embarrassed at having to use a spot of lubricant. Its also important not to only have ejaculation as the goal. Pleasure is a better goal. Being connected is a great pleasure, but rubbing the vagina until it hurts is not a pleasure. A useful website can be found at http://www.sexasnatureintendedit.com/10F/9less_love.html based on the book of the same title by Kristen O Hara. However, don't expect solutions from this book as it is mainly pointing out the errors of men's ways!

More Food and Sex

A scientific viewpoint

(A chapter for the technophiles!)
(See the Glossary for technical word definitions)

Good foods are those that don't cause disease or illness, and contribute to the health of the body. Sometimes a food that is good for one person is bad for another. This is because of genetics. One's body type is determined by a gene which one inherits from one's parents. One's blood type is also determined by a gene which one inherits from one's parents. The blood types are named according to a factor that creates antibodies in the blood; A or B, or O if the blood doesn't carry the antigen to make the antibody. The blood type gene is carried along with many other genes in a chromosome which also carries genes related to health, eye colour, and hair colour.

Genes determine what one can safely eat. There are natural molecules in food called lectins. Lectins are carbohydrate-binding proteins that are neither enzymes nor antibodies. Lectins cause allergy-like reactions. For example a mushroom lectin can cause thrombosis and kidney failure. This what a mushroom lectin looks like (the different colour ribbons are strings of different molecules):

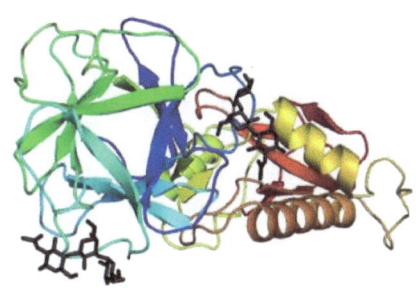

Mushroom Lectin

The different blood types react to different lectins:

In the cereal group, for example, the wheat lectin is different to the rye lectin, and they are both different to rice. Relating this to the blood type means that blood type B cannot eat rye, and blood type O cannot eat wheat, but both type O and type B can eat rice. Similarly blood type O can safely eat chicken but blood type B has to avoid chicken. All the details and lists of foods for each blood type are in the book 'Live Right For your Type' by Dr Peter D'Adamo.

The lectin sensitivity is not always present, and it is not the only reason for immune problems, but it is worth trying the blood type diet for a few months if one is trying to improve health. We feel sexy and attractive if we look good, so a face full of spots is bound to detract from that sexiness. Type B people have been known to struggle with a spotty face for years, but have it completely clear up in a couple of weeks while avoiding tomatoes. The most enjoyment from sex is obtained when one is feeling healthy and fit. Anything that takes one in that direction is a bonus. An added bonus is that weight loss is quite common while following the blood type diet.

Of course, someone will say that they feel fit and well despite eating any and everything. The question is: Do they have a fulfilling sex life at sixty? If not, they might benefit from a change in diet!

Some people react to chemicals in food, and others don't. It depends on the level of nutrients in the liver to antidote the chemicals. Remember that alcohol is a chemical too. Every toxin circulating in the blood has to go through the liver and the kidneys where the body tries to change it from harmful to harmless then filter it out through the urine. Some toxins don't get that far because the body stores the toxin (such as the pesticide DDT) in fat. The brain is 70% fat and some of the toxins end up there. The result is gradual brain death. Lead, mercury, arsenic, and aluminium all affect the brain and the nervous system which ultimately will impair the ability to get satisfaction from sex. These metallic toxins can get into the body through food and water. The group of preservatives called Parabens are toxins too, and have been associated with cancer.

Parabens have been found in breast milk. How good is that for the baby?

All toxins are de-toxified through enzymes, vitamins, and minerals. If one's diet is lacking these nutrients, no matter how healthy one appears to be, eventually the detoxification processes will fail. These same nutrients are used in everyday normal life to make energy so any deficiency will show as a loss of energy, often heard as 'tired all the time'. Alcohol is a toxin that uses vitamin B3 for part of its detoxification but the B3 is also needed to open the gateway for cholesterol to become steroid hormones. These include the sex hormones testosterone, estrogen, and progesterone, as well as cortisol, and vitamin D. Cortisol allows us to cope with stress, and vitamin D protects us from infection and cancer while at the same time building our bones. Naturally, vitamin B3 is not found in junk food.

Food gives us energy, and we need that energy for sex. Being too tired to perform is not good for a relationship!

How does food become energy? Think of lighting a fire – you need fuel, oxygen, and something to get it started. Food is the fuel, oxygen is in the air you breathe, and enzymes are the firelighters. In simple terms the food is broken down to glucose which then provides the energy. Along the way the process uses enzymes to take apart and re-arrange the food molecules. The enzymes, in turn, need vitamins and minerals to perform their job. Enzymes are used because they can operate at low temperatures such as found in a living body, 37 degrees C. A candle flame, by comparison, is several hundred degrees C!

The first step in this chain uses magnesium as a co-factor to activate the enzyme. Strangely, it is magnesium that is most often deficient because it is found in foods which people tend to shy away from; green leaves, nuts, and seeds. Wheatgrass and pumpkin seeds are good sources. At the very end of the energy-from-glucose chain there is one element remaining which, if it can't be safely disposed of, will block the whole cycle with the result that no energy could be produced. That element is hydrogen, and it contains a particle of electricity, the electron. It is the movement of hydrogen and its electron in a special cell called the Mitochondria that actually makes energy, finally combining the hydrogen atoms with oxygen atoms to make water. Remember, H_2O? (The 'H' is Hydrogen, and the 'O' is Oxygen).

During sexual intercourse much energy is expended, and the sweat that runs off the panting body has come from the end of the cycle when hydrogen and oxygen join to make water.

At last, energy – and sex! Well, nearly. You have to breathe too because that is where the oxygen comes from. Your effort at panting for breath is the body doing its best to supply the oxygen by breathing harder and faster.

For some people, this is the source of the problem of no energy. To capture the oxygen which one has just breathed in, one requires hemoglobin in the blood, and that requires iron. Dried beans and dark green leafy vegetables are especially good sources of iron, so is meat. Blood type 'O' seems to be better able to digest and assimilate the nourishment in meat. Blood type 'A' has a tendency to develop arthritis from red meat. Vitamin C increases absorption of iron so it is useful to include fresh vegetables or fruits at every meal. When in Spain I noticed that Spanish locals always have fresh raw onions with their lunchtime salads. Onions are high in vitamin C. At night they had cooked food. However, it might be advisable to avoid raw onions before a romantic date: the smell of onions may not be a sexual turn-on! One little extra step before one can waltz the partner into the boudoir concerns the stomach. The secretions on the inside of the stomach are just as important as the six-pack on the outside. The stomach is a way to the man's heart in more ways than one. The wrong food may cause a heart attack, but also, the stomach secretes acid which makes iron soluble, and secretes a mysterious substance that allows vitamin B12 to be absorbed too. B12 is part of the iron absorption cycle in the intestine. The acid in the stomach originates, indirectly, from the activity of vitamin B3. The excitement and passion under the sheets is never very far removed from the stomach and good eating habits. Like everything else in the body, it is enzymes that control the production of stomach acid. These enzymes need the mineral zinc to activate their function, and zinc needs stomach acid to aid its absorption. In this circular fashion, lack of zinc might be the cause of energy deficiency, tiredness, and no sex.

It is energy that creates satisfying sex at sixty! The food you eat must contain the vitamins and minerals needed by your blood, in order to make energy. Because some food is lacking these essential nutrients one has to add them to one's diet as supplements. The skill is knowing which one to supplement and in what amount. This is the field of the Naturopath trained in Applied-Kinesiology and Clinical Nutrition.

In a Nutshell

Sex is normal and natural but education on the subject is usually in the direction of avoidance of pregnancy rather than satisfaction and enjoyment. Hopefully this book corrects the balance. Better late than never!

Sex is a dynamic urge, created by nature to make sure we reproduce. Fortunately this urge remains even after the reproductive years have passed, i.e. menopause has occurred. By selecting the most suitable foods for one's genetic type and constitution it is possible to be fit and healthy well past one's 60th birthday. In fact it is never too late to reform one's diet for the purpose of getting more satisfaction from sex.

The key elements of the diet are that it must provide a high proportion of vegetables both in cooked and salad form, and that it must match the blood type of the individual. It is also vital that vitamin D3 is supplemented during the cooler months of October to March, with at least 2000 i.u.'s per day of the vitamin.

Practice the vaginal muscle exercises every day for at least 3 months to begin with, and have a partner gently massage the clitoris and G-spot daily. Also massage each other's face, head, and neck every morning – friends will start wondering which health spa you are visiting! Walking is one of the best forms of exercise to increase oxygen in the blood which you need to get satisfaction from sex. Walk as often and as far as you can: It keeps you young and is good for your heart too.

Finally, relax. Sex at sixty is not about achieving a goal, like a mountain to be conquered. The satisfaction of sex at sixty is about feeling passion for one's partner, not just between the sheets but all day and every day. Enjoy it!

References and Credits

Some of the data and images in this study are in the public domain via the internet. The author is grateful to the researchers who made their data freely available. Some are individually acknowledged below.

Green Remedies supply vitamins, minerals, and co-factors in pure-fill capsule form or liquid. Contact: info@greenremedies.com

http://ods.od.nih.gov/factsheets/chromium

http://vitamindcouncil.org Everything about vitamin D.

http://www.dothekegel.com/arnie/index.html Arnold H. Kegel, MD, FACS. Stress Incontinence and Genital Relaxation. CIBA Clinical Symposia, Feb-Mar 1952, Vol. 4, No. 2, pages 35-52

http://incontinet.com/kegelpix.htm More on Kegel exercises.

http://www.slidefinder.net/p/pelvicfloorworkshops2006/32153391

http://en.wikipedia.org/wiki/Clitoris

http://www.womenshealthinwomenshands.org/Anatomy.htm
Images taken from a New View of a Woman's Body, A Fully Illustrative Guide by the Federation of Feminists Women's Health Centres
Drawings by Suzann Gage.

If you like science you can find more online about sex and natural hormones here: http://www.reuniting.info/science/sex_in_the_brain (by Gary Wilson and Marnia Robinson). Also, a study published in 2002 by anthropologist Helen Fisher PhD of Rutgers University: http://www.mcmanweb.com/love_lust.html

http://www.netdoctor.co.uk/sexandrelationships/medicinessex.htm

http://folk.uio.no/utek/projects/lectins.shtml Mushroom Lectin
Research.

P. D'Adamo 'Live Right for Your Type' Comprehensive book by
this author on choosing suitable foods for a healthier life based on an
individual's blood type.

Glossary help
http://www.thefreedictionary.com
Photograph 'Sexy at Sixty, Naturally!' by K Green
Title Page art by HK Art, Da Fen Village, Buji Town, Shenzhen,
Guangdong, China
'Salad' image creator Suat Eman: FreeDigitalPhotos.net
http://www.freedigitalphotos.net/images/view_photog.php?photogid
=151

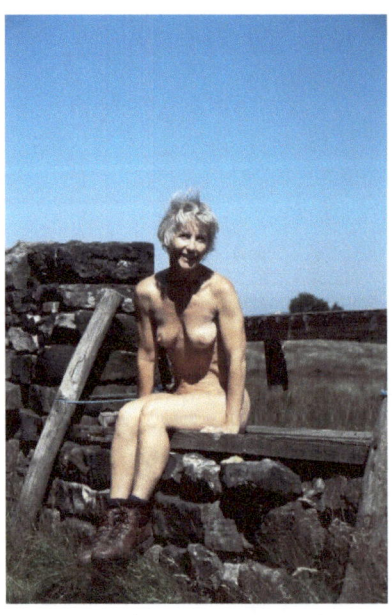

Making the most of English sunshine!

Glossary

Amide:	Containing an amino group, NH2. This is related to ammonia.
Atom:	The smallest unit of a physical substance, having all the characteristics of that substance. Atoms are made from positive, negative, and neutral electric charges. Hydrogen is the smallest and lightest atom having just one negative, and one positive charge, At the other end of the scale Lead is a very large and heavy atom with 82 negative, and 82 positive charges.
Bartholin	Danish anatomist Caspar Bartholin (1655–1738).
Bartholin's glands	Glands located slightly behind and on either side of the opening of the vagina. They secrete mucus to lubricate the vagina.
Calorie:	A unit of energy.
Cardiovascular:	Heart and blood vessels of the heart. Usually refers to disease of these parts through blockage by fat deposits.
Chlorophyll:	Green pigments that are found in plants.
Cholesterol:	A sterol found widely in animal and plant tissues. It is a main component of blood plasma and cell membranes, and it is an important precursor of many steroid hormones (such as the estrogens, testosterone, and cortisol), vitamin D, and bile acids. In vertebrates, cholesterol is manufactured by the liver or absorbed from food in the intestine.
Co-enzyme:	A non-protein organic substance that usually contains a vitamin or mineral and helps to activate an enzyme.
Digestion:.	The process by which food is converted into substances that can be absorbed and assimilated by the body.
Digestive System:	The organs of digestion, including, mouth, stomach, intestine, liver, gall-bladder, pancreas, and colon.
Dopamine	A hormone produced in the brain. Lack of dopamine causes involuntary shaking and loss of muscle control.
Ejaculation	The orgasm of the male that ejects fluid through the penis.
Electron:	The negative charge in an atom of Hydrogen. The number of electrons equals the number of Protons in the nucleus of the atom. Electrons create the current in electricity.
Element:	A substance composed of atoms having the same number of protons in each atom. E.g. A piece of iron is made from many atoms that each have twenty six protons. Elements cannot be reduced to simpler substances by normal chemical means.
Estrogen	A hormone produced in the ovary that creates female characteristics.
Glucose:	The principal circulating sugar in the blood and the major energy source of the body. A simple single molecule sugar.

Hypertension:	Abnormally high blood pressure.
Insulin:	A hormone, secreted in the pancreas, that controls the concentration of glucose in the blood. Insulin deficiency results in diabetes mellitus.
Molecule:	The simplest unit of a chemical compound that can exist. It must contain at least two atoms.
NAD:	Nicotinamide adenine dinucleotide. A co-enzyme that occurs in many living cells and functions as an electron acceptor. NAD is used alternately with NADH as an oxidising or reducing agent in metabolic reactions (giving or receiving hydrogen).
NADPH:	Nicotinamide adenine dinucleotide phosphate, plus hydrogen: a co-enzyme with functions similar to those of NAD.
Nicotinamide:	The amide of nicotinic acid: vitamin B3.
Nucleus:	The bit in the middle. Atoms are mostly empty space, with all the mass or weight of the atom in the middle, the nucleus. This nucleus is balanced by the negative charge (electron) on the outside of the atom.
Nutrition:	The study of food and nourishment, including food composition, dietary guidelines, and the roles that various nutrients have in maintaining health.
Obesity:	Increased body weight caused by excessive accumulation of fat.
Organic compounds:	A compound of carbon. Also includes an element, e.g. hydrogen.
Orgasm:	The peak of sexual excitement, characterised by strong feelings of pleasure and by a series of involuntary contractions of the muscles of the genitals, usually accompanied by the ejaculation of semen by the male.
Oxytocin	A hormone produced in the brain.
Proton:	The positively charged particle in the nucleus of an atom.
Scurvy:	A disease caused by vitamin C deficiency, characterised by bleeding of the gums, rupture of capillaries under the skin, loose teeth, and generalised weakness.
Seminal fluid	The ejaculate from the penis containing sperm cells and prostate fluid.
Skene	Alexander Skene (1837–1900) British gynaecologist who described what became known as Skene's glands.
Skene's Gland	Para-urethral glands, located on the front wall of the vagina, around the lower end of the urethra. They drain into the urethra near the urethral opening.
Smoothies:	a smooth, thick drink made with puréed fresh fruit and yogurt, ice cream, or milk.
Steroid:	Any of a large class of organic compounds having as a basis 17 carbon atoms arranged in four rings fused together.

	Steroids include many biologically important compounds, including cholesterol and other sterols, the sex hormones (such as testosterone and estrogen), bile acids, adrenal hormones, plant alkaloids, and certain forms of vitamins.
Sterol:	A waxy insoluble natural alcohol. Sterols are found in the tissues of animals, plants, fungi, and yeasts and include cholesterol.
Supplements:	Something added to food to improve its quality. Concentrated extracts of food, such as vitamins and minerals, to balance a deficiency in food or diet.
Testosterone	A hormone that is produced in the testes and creates male characteristics. It is also produced in the female and influences sex drive (libido).
Thyroxin:	A hormone, produced by the thyroid gland to regulate metabolism. Thyroxin contains the mineral Iodine.
Urethra	The canal through which urine is discharged from the bladder.
Vasopressin	A hormone produced in the brain that controls urine flow and arterial pressure.
Vegan:	Food that is free of animal ingredients. Vegetable ingredients only. A person who eats this kind of food.
Vitamin:	Any of a group of substances that are essential, in small quantities, for the normal functioning of life in the body.

About the Author

Kenneth G Green ND. HD. MRN.

Kenneth is a Doctor of Homeopathy and Naturopathy (RSA) and a member of the British Naturopathic Association, registered with the General Council and Register of Naturopaths.

He has further qualifications in Bowen Technique, Homeopathy, Nutrition, Kinesiology, Sound Therapy, and Counselling.

Kenneth was formerly resident osteopath and deputy principal at the Savoy Forest Mere Hydro in Hampshire, and manager of therapies at Tyringham Naturopathic Clinic in Buckinghamshire.

Kenneth has been Director of the Cleveland Natural Health Clinic for the past 22 years.

www.ingramcontent.com/pod-product-compliance
Lightning Source LLC
Chambersburg PA
CBHW050820290526
45792CB00001B/201